Dull, aching pain on both sides of the h A feeling of pressure behind the eyes The sensation of tightness at the back (head Tender neck or shoulder muscles	
Sudden pain in the temples, the top of the head or behind your ears Tenderness or swelling to the top, sides, front or back of the head A sore scalp Jaw pain, typically when chewing or talking Visual problems, fatique, fever	Giant Cell Arteritis
Stabbing or burning pain centred over one eye or temple Severe or excruciating pain lasting from a few minutes to a few hours A red and watering eye A drooping or swollen eyelid A blocked or runny nose A shrunken or constricted pupil Sweating	Cluster
Throbbing pain in the forehead or cheeks Facial tenderness or swelling A blocked or runny nose Green or yellow discharge from the nose Earache Fever	Sinus
Throbbing pain on one side of the head Moderate to severe pain Blurred vision, seeing flashing lights or zigzag lines Increased sensitivity to light, smells or loud noises Feeling lightheaded Nausea and/or vomiting	Migraine

EXAMPLE

DATE 25/4/22

TIME

	begin	end	duration		begin	end	duration
1	10:30	12:30	2 hrs	3	19:30		
2	15:10	15:30	20 m	4			

LOCATION

tension	gca	cluster	sinus	migraine	neck
1		23			

SEVERITY

1	2	3	4	5	6	7 ✓	8	9	10

MILD   SEVERE

TRIGGERS

☐ coffee	☐ insomnia	☐ eye strain	☐ smell
☐ alcohol	☐ stress	☐ sickness	☐
☐ medication	☐ bright light	☐ travel	☐
☐ food	☐ pc/tv screen	☑ motion	☐
☐ weather	☐ reading	☐ anxiety	☐
☑ allergies	☐ noise	☐ pms	☐

RELIEF MEASURES

medication	Took 2 painkillers 10 am + 3 pm
sleep/rest	
exercise	Neck massage helped relief pain
Other	

DATE 25/4/12

	begin	end	duration		begin	end	duration
1	wake up. 10 00	12·05	2:15h ① side	3			
2	2000	?	? slp	4			

LOCATION

tension	gca	cluster	sinus	migraine	neck

i — migraine
✓ — neck *evening*

SEVERITY

1	2	3	④	5	6	7	8	9	10
MILD									SEVERE

TRIGGERS

- [ ] coffee
- [x] insomnia
- [x] eye strain ?
- [ ] smell
- [ ] alcohol
- [x] stress ?
- [ ] sickness
- [x] neck pain + shoulder.
- [x] medication ?
- [ ] bright light
- [ ] travel
- [ ]
- [ ] food
- [x] pc/tv screen — evening
- [ ] motion
- [ ]
- [ ] weather
- [x] reading phone
- [ ] anxiety
- [ ]
- [ ] allergies
- [ ] noise
- [ ] pms
- [ ]

RELIEF MEASURES

medication	Migralue x 1 yellow.
sleep/rest	rest - lens chaves
exercise	Pilates .
Other	

DATE	

TIME

	begin	end	duration		begin	end	duration
1				3			
2				4			

LOCATION

tension	gca	cluster	sinus	migraine	neck

SEVERITY

1	2	3	4	5	6	7	8	9	10

MILD   SEVERE

TRIGGERS

☐ coffee	☐ insomnia	☐ eye strain	☐ smell
☐ alcohol	☐ stress	☐ sickness	☐
☐ medication	☐ bright light	☐ travel	☐
☐ food	☐ pc/tv screen	☐ motion	☐
☐ weather	☐ reading	☐ anxiety	☐
☐ allergies	☐ noise	☐ pms	☐

RELIEF MEASURES

medication	
sleep/rest	
exercise	
Other	

	DATE	

TIME

	begin	end	duration		begin	end	duration
1				3			
2				4			

LOCATION

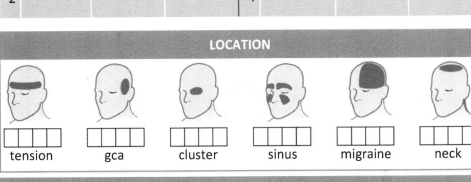

tension	gca	cluster	sinus	migraine	neck

SEVERITY

1	2	3	4	5	6	7	8	9	10

MILD   SEVERE

TRIGGERS

☐ coffee	☐ insomnia	☐ eye strain	☐ smell
☐ alcohol	☐ stress	☐ sickness	☐
☐ medication	☐ bright light	☐ travel	☐
☐ food	☐ pc/tv screen	☐ motion	☐
☐ weather	☐ reading	☐ anxiety	☐
☐ allergies	☐ noise	☐ pms	☐

RELIEF MEASURES

medication	
sleep/rest	
exercise	
Other	

			DATE		

TIME

	begin	end	duration		begin	end	duration
1				3			
2				4			

LOCATION

tension	gca	cluster	sinus	migraine	neck

SEVERITY

1	2	3	4	5	6	7	8	9	10

MILD   SEVERE

TRIGGERS

☐ coffee	☐ insomnia	☐ eye strain	☐ smell
☐ alcohol	☐ stress	☐ sickness	☐
☐ medication	☐ bright light	☐ travel	☐
☐ food	☐ pc/tv screen	☐ motion	☐
☐ weather	☐ reading	☐ anxiety	☐
☐ allergies	☐ noise	☐ pms	☐

RELIEF MEASURES

medication	
sleep/rest	
exercise	
Other	

			DATE	

TIME

	begin	end	duration		begin	end	duration
1				3			
2				4			

LOCATION

tension	gca	cluster	sinus	migraine	neck
☐☐☐☐☐	☐☐☐☐☐	☐☐☐☐☐	☐☐☐☐☐	☐☐☐☐☐	☐☐☐☐

SEVERITY

1	2	3	4	5	6	7	8	9	10
MILD									SEVERE

TRIGGERS

☐ coffee	☐ insomnia	☐ eye strain	☐ smell
☐ alcohol	☐ stress	☐ sickness	☐
☐ medication	☐ bright light	☐ travel	☐
☐ food	☐ pc/tv screen	☐ motion	☐
☐ weather	☐ reading	☐ anxiety	☐
☐ allergies	☐ noise	☐ pms	☐

RELIEF MEASURES

medication	
sleep/rest	
exercise	
Other	

	DATE	

TIME

	begin	end	duration		begin	end	duration
1				3			
2				4			

LOCATION

tension	gca	cluster	sinus	migraine	neck

SEVERITY

1	2	3	4	5	6	7	8	9	10

MILD   SEVERE

TRIGGERS

☐ coffee	☐ insomnia	☐ eye strain	☐ smell
☐ alcohol	☐ stress	☐ sickness	☐
☐ medication	☐ bright light	☐ travel	☐
☐ food	☐ pc/tv screen	☐ motion	☐
☐ weather	☐ reading	☐ anxiety	☐
☐ allergies	☐ noise	☐ pms	☐

RELIEF MEASURES

medication	
sleep/rest	
exercise	
Other	

DATE	

TIME

	begin	end	duration		begin	end	duration
1				3			
2				4			

LOCATION

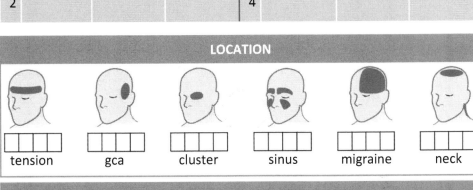

tension	gca	cluster	sinus	migraine	neck

SEVERITY

1	2	3	4	5	6	7	8	9	10

MILD   SEVERE

TRIGGERS

☐ coffee	☐ insomnia	☐ eye strain	☐ smell
☐ alcohol	☐ stress	☐ sickness	☐
☐ medication	☐ bright light	☐ travel	☐
☐ food	☐ pc/tv screen	☐ motion	☐
☐ weather	☐ reading	☐ anxiety	☐
☐ allergies	☐ noise	☐ pms	☐

RELIEF MEASURES

medication	
sleep/rest	
exercise	
Other	

	DATE	

TIME

	begin	end	duration		begin	end	duration
1				3			
2				4			

LOCATION

tension	gca	cluster	sinus	migraine	neck

SEVERITY

1	2	3	4	5	6	7	8	9	10

MILD   SEVERE

TRIGGERS

☐ coffee	☐ insomnia	☐ eye strain	☐ smell
☐ alcohol	☐ stress	☐ sickness	☐
☐ medication	☐ bright light	☐ travel	☐
☐ food	☐ pc/tv screen	☐ motion	☐
☐ weather	☐ reading	☐ anxiety	☐
☐ allergies	☐ noise	☐ pms	☐

RELIEF MEASURES

medication	
sleep/rest	
exercise	
Other	

DATE	

TIME

	begin	end	duration		begin	end	duration
1				3			
2				4			

LOCATION

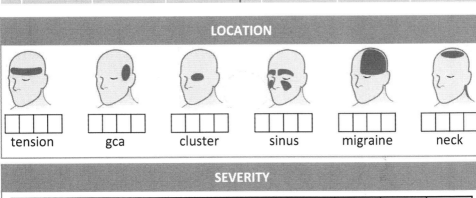

tension	gca	cluster	sinus	migraine	neck

SEVERITY

1	2	3	4	5	6	7	8	9	10

MILD   SEVERE

TRIGGERS

☐ coffee	☐ insomnia	☐ eye strain	☐ smell
☐ alcohol	☐ stress	☐ sickness	☐
☐ medication	☐ bright light	☐ travel	☐
☐ food	☐ pc/tv screen	☐ motion	☐
☐ weather	☐ reading	☐ anxiety	☐
☐ allergies	☐ noise	☐ pms	☐

RELIEF MEASURES

medication	
sleep/rest	
exercise	
Other	

	DATE	

TIME

	begin	end	duration		begin	end	duration
1				3			
2				4			

LOCATION

tension	gca	cluster	sinus	migraine	neck

SEVERITY

1	2	3	4	5	6	7	8	9	10

MILD   SEVERE

TRIGGERS

☐ coffee	☐ insomnia	☐ eye strain	☐ smell
☐ alcohol	☐ stress	☐ sickness	☐
☐ medication	☐ bright light	☐ travel	☐
☐ food	☐ pc/tv screen	☐ motion	☐
☐ weather	☐ reading	☐ anxiety	☐
☐ allergies	☐ noise	☐ pms	☐

RELIEF MEASURES

medication	
sleep/rest	
exercise	
Other	

DATE	

TIME

	begin	end	duration		begin	end	duration
1				3			
2				4			

LOCATION

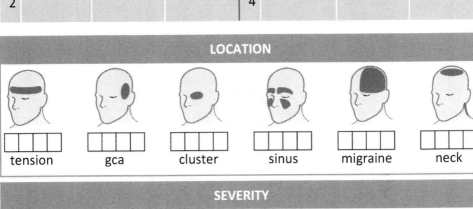

tension	gca	cluster	sinus	migraine	neck

SEVERITY

1	2	3	4	5	6	7	8	9	10

MILD   SEVERE

TRIGGERS

☐ coffee	☐ insomnia	☐ eye strain	☐ smell
☐ alcohol	☐ stress	☐ sickness	☐
☐ medication	☐ bright light	☐ travel	☐
☐ food	☐ pc/tv screen	☐ motion	☐
☐ weather	☐ reading	☐ anxiety	☐
☐ allergies	☐ noise	☐ pms	☐

RELIEF MEASURES

medication	
sleep/rest	
exercise	
Other	

	DATE	

TIME

	begin	end	duration		begin	end	duration
1				3			
2				4			

LOCATION

tension	gca	cluster	sinus	migraine	neck

SEVERITY

1	2	3	4	5	6	7	8	9	10

MILD   SEVERE

TRIGGERS

☐ coffee	☐ insomnia	☐ eye strain	☐ smell
☐ alcohol	☐ stress	☐ sickness	☐
☐ medication	☐ bright light	☐ travel	☐
☐ food	☐ pc/tv screen	☐ motion	☐
☐ weather	☐ reading	☐ anxiety	☐
☐ allergies	☐ noise	☐ pms	☐

RELIEF MEASURES

medication	
sleep/rest	
exercise	
Other	

	DATE		

TIME

	begin	end	duration		begin	end	duration
1				3			
2				4			

LOCATION

tension	gca	cluster	sinus	migraine	neck

SEVERITY

1	2	3	4	5	6	7	8	9	10
MILD									SEVERE

TRIGGERS

☐ coffee	☐ insomnia	☐ eye strain	☐ smell
☐ alcohol	☐ stress	☐ sickness	☐
☐ medication	☐ bright light	☐ travel	☐
☐ food	☐ pc/tv screen	☐ motion	☐
☐ weather	☐ reading	☐ anxiety	☐
☐ allergies	☐ noise	☐ pms	☐

RELIEF MEASURES

medication	
sleep/rest	
exercise	
Other	

DATE	

TIME

	begin	end	duration		begin	end	duration
1				3			
2				4			

LOCATION

tension	gca	cluster	sinus	migraine	neck

SEVERITY

1	2	3	4	5	6	7	8	9	10

MILD   SEVERE

TRIGGERS

☐ coffee	☐ insomnia	☐ eye strain	☐ smell
☐ alcohol	☐ stress	☐ sickness	☐
☐ medication	☐ bright light	☐ travel	☐
☐ food	☐ pc/tv screen	☐ motion	☐
☐ weather	☐ reading	☐ anxiety	☐
☐ allergies	☐ noise	☐ pms	☐

RELIEF MEASURES

medication	
sleep/rest	
exercise	
Other	

DATE	

TIME

	begin	end	duration		begin	end	duration
1				3			
2				4			

LOCATION

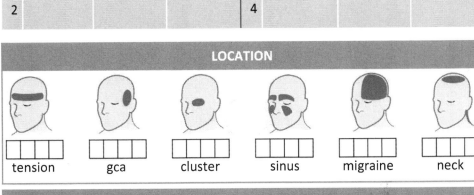

tension	gca	cluster	sinus	migraine	neck

SEVERITY

1	2	3	4	5	6	7	8	9	10

MILD   SEVERE

TRIGGERS

☐ coffee	☐ insomnia	☐ eye strain	☐ smell
☐ alcohol	☐ stress	☐ sickness	☐
☐ medication	☐ bright light	☐ travel	☐
☐ food	☐ pc/tv screen	☐ motion	☐
☐ weather	☐ reading	☐ anxiety	☐
☐ allergies	☐ noise	☐ pms	☐

RELIEF MEASURES

medication	
sleep/rest	
exercise	
Other	

		DATE				

TIME

	begin	end	duration		begin	end	duration
1				3			
2				4			

LOCATION

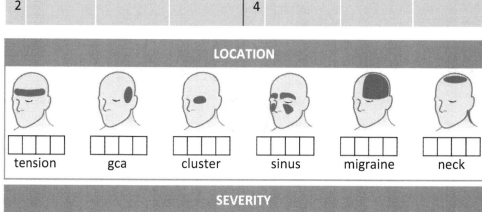

tension	gca	cluster	sinus	migraine	neck
☐☐☐☐	☐☐☐☐	☐☐☐☐	☐☐☐☐	☐☐☐☐	☐☐☐☐

SEVERITY

1	2	3	4	5	6	7	8	9	10
MILD									SEVERE

TRIGGERS

☐ coffee	☐ insomnia	☐ eye strain	☐ smell
☐ alcohol	☐ stress	☐ sickness	☐
☐ medication	☐ bright light	☐ travel	☐
☐ food	☐ pc/tv screen	☐ motion	☐
☐ weather	☐ reading	☐ anxiety	☐
☐ allergies	☐ noise	☐ pms	☐

RELIEF MEASURES

medication	
sleep/rest	
exercise	
Other	

		DATE	

TIME

	begin	end	duration		begin	end	duration
1				3			
2				4			

LOCATION

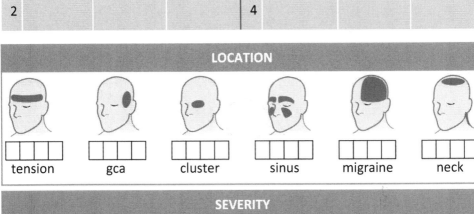

tension	gca	cluster	sinus	migraine	neck

SEVERITY

1	2	3	4	5	6	7	8	9	10

MILD   SEVERE

TRIGGERS

☐ coffee	☐ insomnia	☐ eye strain	☐ smell
☐ alcohol	☐ stress	☐ sickness	☐
☐ medication	☐ bright light	☐ travel	☐
☐ food	☐ pc/tv screen	☐ motion	☐
☐ weather	☐ reading	☐ anxiety	☐
☐ allergies	☐ noise	☐ pms	☐

RELIEF MEASURES

medication	
sleep/rest	
exercise	
Other	

	DATE	

TIME

	begin	end	duration		begin	end	duration
1				3			
2				4			

LOCATION

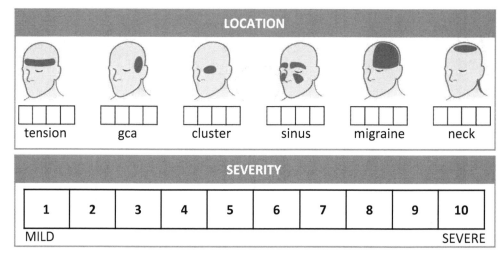

tension	gca	cluster	sinus	migraine	neck

SEVERITY

1	2	3	4	5	6	7	8	9	10

MILD   SEVERE

TRIGGERS

☐ coffee	☐ insomnia	☐ eye strain	☐ smell
☐ alcohol	☐ stress	☐ sickness	☐
☐ medication	☐ bright light	☐ travel	☐
☐ food	☐ pc/tv screen	☐ motion	☐
☐ weather	☐ reading	☐ anxiety	☐
☐ allergies	☐ noise	☐ pms	☐

RELIEF MEASURES

medication	
sleep/rest	
exercise	
Other	

	DATE		

TIME

	begin	end	duration		begin	end	duration
1				3			
2				4			

LOCATION

tension	gca	cluster	sinus	migraine	neck

SEVERITY

1	2	3	4	5	6	7	8	9	10

MILD   SEVERE

TRIGGERS

☐ coffee	☐ insomnia	☐ eye strain	☐ smell
☐ alcohol	☐ stress	☐ sickness	☐
☐ medication	☐ bright light	☐ travel	☐
☐ food	☐ pc/tv screen	☐ motion	☐
☐ weather	☐ reading	☐ anxiety	☐
☐ allergies	☐ noise	☐ pms	☐

RELIEF MEASURES

medication	
sleep/rest	
exercise	
Other	

DATE	

TIME

	begin	end	duration		begin	end	duration
1				3			
2				4			

LOCATION

tension	gca	cluster	sinus	migraine	neck

SEVERITY

1	2	3	4	5	6	7	8	9	10

MILD   SEVERE

TRIGGERS

☐ coffee	☐ insomnia	☐ eye strain	☐ smell
☐ alcohol	☐ stress	☐ sickness	☐
☐ medication	☐ bright light	☐ travel	☐
☐ food	☐ pc/tv screen	☐ motion	☐
☐ weather	☐ reading	☐ anxiety	☐
☐ allergies	☐ noise	☐ pms	☐

RELIEF MEASURES

medication	
sleep/rest	
exercise	
Other	

	DATE	

TIME

	begin	end	duration		begin	end	duration
1				3			
2				4			

LOCATION

tension	gca	cluster	sinus	migraine	neck

SEVERITY

1	2	3	4	5	6	7	8	9	10

MILD   SEVERE

TRIGGERS

☐ coffee	☐ insomnia	☐ eye strain	☐ smell
☐ alcohol	☐ stress	☐ sickness	☐
☐ medication	☐ bright light	☐ travel	☐
☐ food	☐ pc/tv screen	☐ motion	☐
☐ weather	☐ reading	☐ anxiety	☐
☐ allergies	☐ noise	☐ pms	☐

RELIEF MEASURES

medication	
sleep/rest	
exercise	
Other	

			DATE			

TIME

	begin	end	duration		begin	end	duration
1				3			
2				4			

LOCATION

tension	gca	cluster	sinus	migraine	neck

SEVERITY

1	2	3	4	5	6	7	8	9	10

MILD   SEVERE

TRIGGERS

- ☐ coffee
- ☐ alcohol
- ☐ medication
- ☐ food
- ☐ weather
- ☐ allergies
- ☐ insomnia
- ☐ stress
- ☐ bright light
- ☐ pc/tv screen
- ☐ reading
- ☐ noise
- ☐ eye strain
- ☐ sickness
- ☐ travel
- ☐ motion
- ☐ anxiety
- ☐ pms
- ☐ smell
- ☐
- ☐
- ☐
- ☐
- ☐

RELIEF MEASURES

medication	
sleep/rest	
exercise	
Other	

	DATE	

TIME

	begin	end	duration		begin	end	duration
1				3			
2				4			

LOCATION

tension	gca	cluster	sinus	migraine	neck

SEVERITY

1	2	3	4	5	6	7	8	9	10

MILD   SEVERE

TRIGGERS

☐ coffee	☐ insomnia	☐ eye strain	☐ smell
☐ alcohol	☐ stress	☐ sickness	☐
☐ medication	☐ bright light	☐ travel	☐
☐ food	☐ pc/tv screen	☐ motion	☐
☐ weather	☐ reading	☐ anxiety	☐
☐ allergies	☐ noise	☐ pms	☐

RELIEF MEASURES

medication	
sleep/rest	
exercise	
Other	

DATE	

TIME

	begin	end	duration		begin	end	duration
1				3			
2				4			

LOCATION

tension	gca	cluster	sinus	migraine	neck
☐☐☐☐	☐☐☐☐	☐☐☐☐	☐☐☐☐	☐☐☐☐	☐☐☐☐

SEVERITY

1	2	3	4	5	6	7	8	9	10

MILD   SEVERE

TRIGGERS

☐ coffee	☐ insomnia	☐ eye strain	☐ smell
☐ alcohol	☐ stress	☐ sickness	☐
☐ medication	☐ bright light	☐ travel	☐
☐ food	☐ pc/tv screen	☐ motion	☐
☐ weather	☐ reading	☐ anxiety	☐
☐ allergies	☐ noise	☐ pms	☐

RELIEF MEASURES

medication	
sleep/rest	
exercise	
Other	

	DATE	

TIME

	begin	end	duration		begin	end	duration
1				3			
2				4			

LOCATION

tension	gca	cluster	sinus	migraine	neck

SEVERITY

1	2	3	4	5	6	7	8	9	10

MILD   SEVERE

TRIGGERS

☐ coffee	☐ insomnia	☐ eye strain	☐ smell
☐ alcohol	☐ stress	☐ sickness	☐
☐ medication	☐ bright light	☐ travel	☐
☐ food	☐ pc/tv screen	☐ motion	☐
☐ weather	☐ reading	☐ anxiety	☐
☐ allergies	☐ noise	☐ pms	☐

RELIEF MEASURES

medication	
sleep/rest	
exercise	
Other	

DATE	

TIME

	begin	end	duration		begin	end	duration
1				3			
2				4			

LOCATION

tension	gca	cluster	sinus	migraine	neck
☐☐☐☐	☐☐☐☐	☐☐☐☐	☐☐☐☐	☐☐☐☐	☐☐☐☐

SEVERITY

1	2	3	4	5	6	7	8	9	10

MILD   SEVERE

TRIGGERS

☐ coffee	☐ insomnia	☐ eye strain	☐ smell
☐ alcohol	☐ stress	☐ sickness	☐
☐ medication	☐ bright light	☐ travel	☐
☐ food	☐ pc/tv screen	☐ motion	☐
☐ weather	☐ reading	☐ anxiety	☐
☐ allergies	☐ noise	☐ pms	☐

RELIEF MEASURES

medication	
sleep/rest	
exercise	
Other	

	DATE	

TIME

	begin	end	duration		begin	end	duration
1				3			
2				4			

LOCATION

tension	gca	cluster	sinus	migraine	neck
☐☐☐☐☐	☐☐☐☐☐	☐☐☐☐☐	☐☐☐☐☐	☐☐☐☐☐	☐☐☐☐☐

SEVERITY

1	2	3	4	5	6	7	8	9	10

MILD   SEVERE

TRIGGERS

☐ coffee	☐ insomnia	☐ eye strain	☐ smell
☐ alcohol	☐ stress	☐ sickness	☐
☐ medication	☐ bright light	☐ travel	☐
☐ food	☐ pc/tv screen	☐ motion	☐
☐ weather	☐ reading	☐ anxiety	☐
☐ allergies	☐ noise	☐ pms	☐

RELIEF MEASURES

medication	
sleep/rest	
exercise	
Other	

			DATE			

TIME

	begin	end	duration		begin	end	duration
1				3			
2				4			

LOCATION

tension	gca	cluster	sinus	migraine	neck

SEVERITY

1	2	3	4	5	6	7	8	9	10

MILD   SEVERE

TRIGGERS

☐ coffee	☐ insomnia	☐ eye strain	☐ smell
☐ alcohol	☐ stress	☐ sickness	☐
☐ medication	☐ bright light	☐ travel	☐
☐ food	☐ pc/tv screen	☐ motion	☐
☐ weather	☐ reading	☐ anxiety	☐
☐ allergies	☐ noise	☐ pms	☐

RELIEF MEASURES

medication	
sleep/rest	
exercise	
Other	

DATE	

TIME

	begin	end	duration		begin	end	duration
1				3			
2				4			

LOCATION

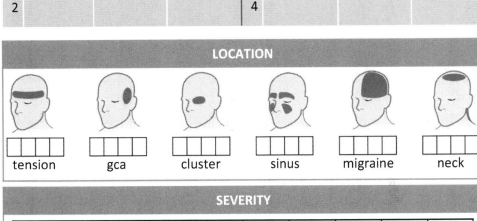

tension	gca	cluster	sinus	migraine	neck

SEVERITY

1	2	3	4	5	6	7	8	9	10

MILD   SEVERE

TRIGGERS

☐ coffee	☐ insomnia	☐ eye strain	☐ smell
☐ alcohol	☐ stress	☐ sickness	☐
☐ medication	☐ bright light	☐ travel	☐
☐ food	☐ pc/tv screen	☐ motion	☐
☐ weather	☐ reading	☐ anxiety	☐
☐ allergies	☐ noise	☐ pms	☐

RELIEF MEASURES

medication	
sleep/rest	
exercise	
Other	

		DATE	

TIME

	begin	end	duration		begin	end	duration
1				3			
2				4			

LOCATION

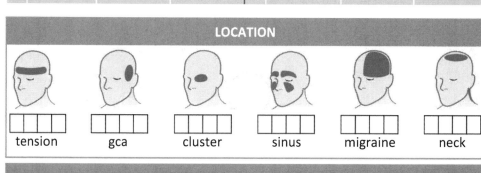

tension	gca	cluster	sinus	migraine	neck

SEVERITY

1	2	3	4	5	6	7	8	9	10

MILD   SEVERE

TRIGGERS

☐ coffee	☐ insomnia	☐ eye strain	☐ smell
☐ alcohol	☐ stress	☐ sickness	☐
☐ medication	☐ bright light	☐ travel	☐
☐ food	☐ pc/tv screen	☐ motion	☐
☐ weather	☐ reading	☐ anxiety	☐
☐ allergies	☐ noise	☐ pms	☐

RELIEF MEASURES

medication	
sleep/rest	
exercise	
Other	

DATE	

TIME

	begin	end	duration		begin	end	duration
1				3			
2				4			

LOCATION

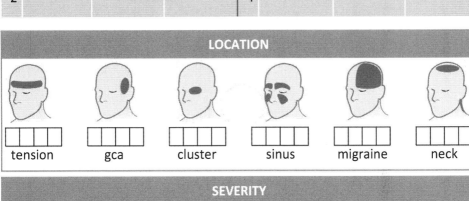

tension	gca	cluster	sinus	migraine	neck

SEVERITY

1	2	3	4	5	6	7	8	9	10

MILD   SEVERE

TRIGGERS

☐ coffee	☐ insomnia	☐ eye strain	☐ smell
☐ alcohol	☐ stress	☐ sickness	☐
☐ medication	☐ bright light	☐ travel	☐
☐ food	☐ pc/tv screen	☐ motion	☐
☐ weather	☐ reading	☐ anxiety	☐
☐ allergies	☐ noise	☐ pms	☐

RELIEF MEASURES

medication	
sleep/rest	
exercise	
Other	

	DATE	

TIME

	begin	end	duration		begin	end	duration
1				3			
2				4			

LOCATION

tension	gca	cluster	sinus	migraine	neck

SEVERITY

1	2	3	4	5	6	7	8	9	10

MILD   SEVERE

TRIGGERS

☐ coffee	☐ insomnia	☐ eye strain	☐ smell
☐ alcohol	☐ stress	☐ sickness	☐
☐ medication	☐ bright light	☐ travel	☐
☐ food	☐ pc/tv screen	☐ motion	☐
☐ weather	☐ reading	☐ anxiety	☐
☐ allergies	☐ noise	☐ pms	☐

RELIEF MEASURES

medication	
sleep/rest	
exercise	
Other	

	DATE	

TIME

	begin	end	duration		begin	end	duration
1				3			
2				4			

LOCATION

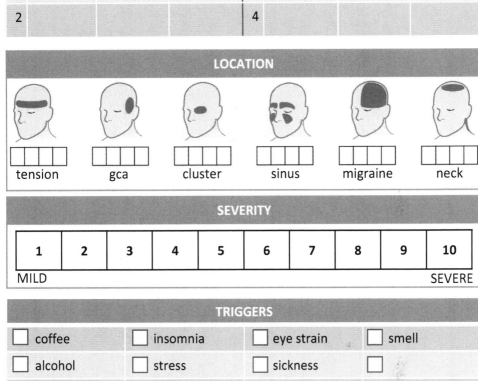

tension	gca	cluster	sinus	migraine	neck

SEVERITY

1	2	3	4	5	6	7	8	9	10

MILD   SEVERE

TRIGGERS

☐ coffee	☐ insomnia	☐ eye strain	☐ smell
☐ alcohol	☐ stress	☐ sickness	☐
☐ medication	☐ bright light	☐ travel	☐
☐ food	☐ pc/tv screen	☐ motion	☐
☐ weather	☐ reading	☐ anxiety	☐
☐ allergies	☐ noise	☐ pms	☐

RELIEF MEASURES

medication	
sleep/rest	
exercise	
Other	

	DATE	

TIME

	begin	end	duration		begin	end	duration
1				3			
2				4			

LOCATION

tension	gca	cluster	sinus	migraine	neck

SEVERITY

1	2	3	4	5	6	7	8	9	10

MILD   SEVERE

TRIGGERS

☐ coffee	☐ insomnia	☐ eye strain	☐ smell
☐ alcohol	☐ stress	☐ sickness	☐
☐ medication	☐ bright light	☐ travel	☐
☐ food	☐ pc/tv screen	☐ motion	☐
☐ weather	☐ reading	☐ anxiety	☐
☐ allergies	☐ noise	☐ pms	☐

RELIEF MEASURES

medication	
sleep/rest	
exercise	
Other	

	DATE	

TIME

	begin	end	duration		begin	end	duration
1				3			
2				4			

LOCATION

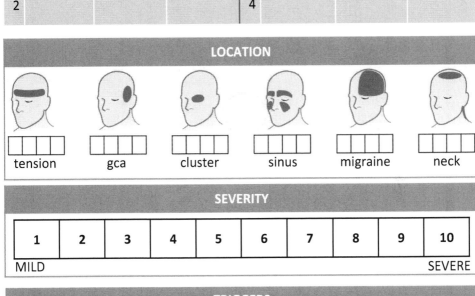

tension	gca	cluster	sinus	migraine	neck
▢▢▢▢	▢▢▢▢	▢▢▢▢	▢▢▢▢	▢▢▢▢	▢▢▢▢

SEVERITY

1	2	3	4	5	6	7	8	9	10

MILD   SEVERE

TRIGGERS

☐ coffee	☐ insomnia	☐ eye strain	☐ smell
☐ alcohol	☐ stress	☐ sickness	☐
☐ medication	☐ bright light	☐ travel	☐
☐ food	☐ pc/tv screen	☐ motion	☐
☐ weather	☐ reading	☐ anxiety	☐
☐ allergies	☐ noise	☐ pms	☐

RELIEF MEASURES

medication	
sleep/rest	
exercise	
Other	

TIME

	begin	end	duration		begin	end	duration
1				3			
2				4			

LOCATION

tension	gca	cluster	sinus	migraine	neck

SEVERITY

1	2	3	4	5	6	7	8	9	10

MILD   SEVERE

TRIGGERS

☐ coffee	☐ insomnia	☐ eye strain	☐ smell
☐ alcohol	☐ stress	☐ sickness	☐
☐ medication	☐ bright light	☐ travel	☐
☐ food	☐ pc/tv screen	☐ motion	☐
☐ weather	☐ reading	☐ anxiety	☐
☐ allergies	☐ noise	☐ pms	☐

RELIEF MEASURES

medication	
sleep/rest	
exercise	
Other	

	DATE						

TIME

	begin	end	duration		begin	end	duration
1				3			
2				4			

LOCATION

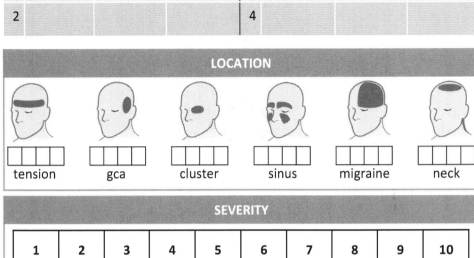

tension	gca	cluster	sinus	migraine	neck

SEVERITY

1	2	3	4	5	6	7	8	9	10
MILD									SEVERE

TRIGGERS

☐ coffee	☐ insomnia	☐ eye strain	☐ smell
☐ alcohol	☐ stress	☐ sickness	☐
☐ medication	☐ bright light	☐ travel	☐
☐ food	☐ pc/tv screen	☐ motion	☐
☐ weather	☐ reading	☐ anxiety	☐
☐ allergies	☐ noise	☐ pms	☐

RELIEF MEASURES

medication	
sleep/rest	
exercise	
Other	

		DATE					

TIME

	begin	end	duration		begin	end	duration
1				3			
2				4			

LOCATION

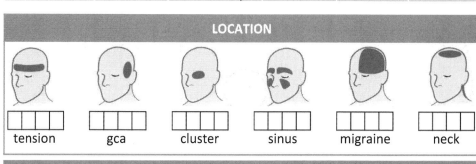

tension	gca	cluster	sinus	migraine	neck

SEVERITY

1	2	3	4	5	6	7	8	9	10

MILD   SEVERE

TRIGGERS

☐ coffee	☐ insomnia	☐ eye strain	☐ smell
☐ alcohol	☐ stress	☐ sickness	☐
☐ medication	☐ bright light	☐ travel	☐
☐ food	☐ pc/tv screen	☐ motion	☐
☐ weather	☐ reading	☐ anxiety	☐
☐ allergies	☐ noise	☐ pms	☐

RELIEF MEASURES

medication	
sleep/rest	
exercise	
Other	

	DATE	

TIME

	begin	end	duration		begin	end	duration
1				3			
2				4			

LOCATION

tension	gca	cluster	sinus	migraine	neck

SEVERITY

1	2	3	4	5	6	7	8	9	10

MILD   SEVERE

TRIGGERS

☐ coffee	☐ insomnia	☐ eye strain	☐ smell
☐ alcohol	☐ stress	☐ sickness	☐
☐ medication	☐ bright light	☐ travel	☐
☐ food	☐ pc/tv screen	☐ motion	☐
☐ weather	☐ reading	☐ anxiety	☐
☐ allergies	☐ noise	☐ pms	☐

RELIEF MEASURES

medication	
sleep/rest	
exercise	
Other	

TIME

	begin	end	duration		begin	end	duration
1				3			
2				4			

LOCATION

tension	gca	cluster	sinus	migraine	neck

SEVERITY

1	2	3	4	5	6	7	8	9	10

MILD   SEVERE

TRIGGERS

☐ coffee	☐ insomnia	☐ eye strain	☐ smell
☐ alcohol	☐ stress	☐ sickness	☐
☐ medication	☐ bright light	☐ travel	☐
☐ food	☐ pc/tv screen	☐ motion	☐
☐ weather	☐ reading	☐ anxiety	☐
☐ allergies	☐ noise	☐ pms	☐

RELIEF MEASURES

medication	
sleep/rest	
exercise	
Other	

	DATE	

TIME

	begin	end	duration		begin	end	duration
1				3			
2				4			

LOCATION

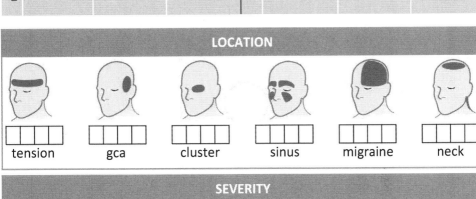

tension	gca	cluster	sinus	migraine	neck

SEVERITY

1	2	3	4	5	6	7	8	9	10

MILD   SEVERE

TRIGGERS

☐ coffee	☐ insomnia	☐ eye strain	☐ smell
☐ alcohol	☐ stress	☐ sickness	☐
☐ medication	☐ bright light	☐ travel	☐
☐ food	☐ pc/tv screen	☐ motion	☐
☐ weather	☐ reading	☐ anxiety	☐
☐ allergies	☐ noise	☐ pms	☐

RELIEF MEASURES

medication	
sleep/rest	
exercise	
Other	

DATE	

TIME

	begin	end	duration		begin	end	duration
1				3			
2				4			

LOCATION

tension	gca	cluster	sinus	migraine	neck
☐☐☐☐	☐☐☐☐	☐☐☐☐	☐☐☐☐	☐☐☐☐	☐☐☐☐

SEVERITY

1	2	3	4	5	6	7	8	9	10

MILD   SEVERE

TRIGGERS

☐ coffee	☐ insomnia	☐ eye strain	☐ smell
☐ alcohol	☐ stress	☐ sickness	☐
☐ medication	☐ bright light	☐ travel	☐
☐ food	☐ pc/tv screen	☐ motion	☐
☐ weather	☐ reading	☐ anxiety	☐
☐ allergies	☐ noise	☐ pms	☐

RELIEF MEASURES

medication	
sleep/rest	
exercise	
Other	

	DATE	

TIME

	begin	end	duration		begin	end	duration
1				3			
2				4			

LOCATION

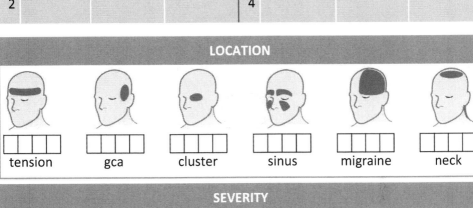

tension	gca	cluster	sinus	migraine	neck
☐☐☐☐	☐☐☐☐	☐☐☐☐	☐☐☐☐	☐☐☐☐	☐☐☐☐

SEVERITY

1	2	3	4	5	6	7	8	9	10

MILD   SEVERE

TRIGGERS

☐ coffee	☐ insomnia	☐ eye strain	☐ smell
☐ alcohol	☐ stress	☐ sickness	☐
☐ medication	☐ bright light	☐ travel	☐
☐ food	☐ pc/tv screen	☐ motion	☐
☐ weather	☐ reading	☐ anxiety	☐
☐ allergies	☐ noise	☐ pms	☐

RELIEF MEASURES

medication	
sleep/rest	
exercise	
Other	

	DATE	

TIME

	begin	end	duration		begin	end	duration
1				3			
2				4			

LOCATION

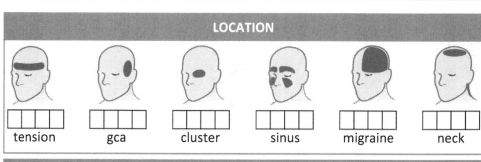

tension	gca	cluster	sinus	migraine	neck

SEVERITY

1	2	3	4	5	6	7	8	9	10

MILD   SEVERE

TRIGGERS

☐ coffee	☐ insomnia	☐ eye strain	☐ smell
☐ alcohol	☐ stress	☐ sickness	☐
☐ medication	☐ bright light	☐ travel	☐
☐ food	☐ pc/tv screen	☐ motion	☐
☐ weather	☐ reading	☐ anxiety	☐
☐ allergies	☐ noise	☐ pms	☐

RELIEF MEASURES

medication	
sleep/rest	
exercise	
Other	

	DATE		

TIME

	begin	end	duration		begin	end	duration
1				3			
2				4			

LOCATION

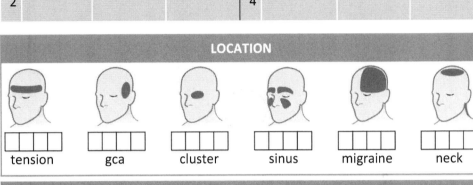

tension	gca	cluster	sinus	migraine	neck

SEVERITY

1	2	3	4	5	6	7	8	9	10

MILD   SEVERE

TRIGGERS

☐ coffee	☐ insomnia	☐ eye strain	☐ smell
☐ alcohol	☐ stress	☐ sickness	☐
☐ medication	☐ bright light	☐ travel	☐
☐ food	☐ pc/tv screen	☐ motion	☐
☐ weather	☐ reading	☐ anxiety	☐
☐ allergies	☐ noise	☐ pms	☐

RELIEF MEASURES

medication	
sleep/rest	
exercise	
Other	

DATE	

TIME

	begin	end	duration		begin	end	duration
1				3			
2				4			

LOCATION

tension	gca	cluster	sinus	migraine	neck
☐☐☐☐	☐☐☐☐	☐☐☐☐	☐☐☐☐	☐☐☐☐☐	☐☐☐☐

SEVERITY

1	2	3	4	5	6	7	8	9	10

MILD   SEVERE

TRIGGERS

☐ coffee	☐ insomnia	☐ eye strain	☐ smell
☐ alcohol	☐ stress	☐ sickness	☐
☐ medication	☐ bright light	☐ travel	☐
☐ food	☐ pc/tv screen	☐ motion	☐
☐ weather	☐ reading	☐ anxiety	☐
☐ allergies	☐ noise	☐ pms	☐

RELIEF MEASURES

medication	
sleep/rest	
exercise	
Other	

DATE	

TIME

	begin	end	duration		begin	end	duration
1				3			
2				4			

LOCATION

tension	gca	cluster	sinus	migraine	neck
☐☐☐☐	☐☐☐☐	☐☐☐☐	☐☐☐☐	☐☐☐☐	☐☐☐

SEVERITY

1	2	3	4	5	6	7	8	9	10
MILD									SEVERE

TRIGGERS

☐ coffee	☐ insomnia	☐ eye strain	☐ smell
☐ alcohol	☐ stress	☐ sickness	☐
☐ medication	☐ bright light	☐ travel	☐
☐ food	☐ pc/tv screen	☐ motion	☐
☐ weather	☐ reading	☐ anxiety	☐
☐ allergies	☐ noise	☐ pms	☐

RELIEF MEASURES

medication	
sleep/rest	
exercise	
Other	

TIME

	begin	end	duration		begin	end	duration
1				3			
2				4			

LOCATION

| tension | gca | cluster | sinus | migraine | neck |

SEVERITY

1	2	3	4	5	6	7	8	9	10

MILD   SEVERE

TRIGGERS

☐ coffee	☐ insomnia	☐ eye strain	☐ smell
☐ alcohol	☐ stress	☐ sickness	☐
☐ medication	☐ bright light	☐ travel	☐
☐ food	☐ pc/tv screen	☐ motion	☐
☐ weather	☐ reading	☐ anxiety	☐
☐ allergies	☐ noise	☐ pms	☐

RELIEF MEASURES

medication	
sleep/rest	
exercise	
Other	

	DATE						

TIME

	begin	end	duration		begin	end	duration
1				3			
2				4			

LOCATION

tension	gca	cluster	sinus	migraine	neck

SEVERITY

1	2	3	4	5	6	7	8	9	10

MILD · SEVERE

TRIGGERS

☐ coffee	☐ insomnia	☐ eye strain	☐ smell
☐ alcohol	☐ stress	☐ sickness	☐
☐ medication	☐ bright light	☐ travel	☐
☐ food	☐ pc/tv screen	☐ motion	☐
☐ weather	☐ reading	☐ anxiety	☐
☐ allergies	☐ noise	☐ pms	☐

RELIEF MEASURES

medication	
sleep/rest	
exercise	
Other	

	DATE		

TIME

	begin	end	duration		begin	end	duration
1				3			
2				4			

LOCATION

tension	gca	cluster	sinus	migraine	neck

SEVERITY

1	2	3	4	5	6	7	8	9	10

MILD   SEVERE

TRIGGERS

☐ coffee	☐ insomnia	☐ eye strain	☐ smell
☐ alcohol	☐ stress	☐ sickness	☐
☐ medication	☐ bright light	☐ travel	☐
☐ food	☐ pc/tv screen	☐ motion	☐
☐ weather	☐ reading	☐ anxiety	☐
☐ allergies	☐ noise	☐ pms	☐

RELIEF MEASURES

medication	
sleep/rest	
exercise	
Other	

DATE	

TIME

	begin	end	duration		begin	end	duration
1				3			
2				4			

LOCATION

tension	gca	cluster	sinus	migraine	neck

SEVERITY

1	2	3	4	5	6	7	8	9	10

MILD   SEVERE

TRIGGERS

coffee	insomnia	eye strain	smell
alcohol	stress	sickness	
medication	bright light	travel	
food	pc/tv screen	motion	
weather	reading	anxiety	
allergies	noise	pms	

RELIEF MEASURES

medication	
sleep/rest	
exercise	
Other	

	DATE	

TIME

	begin	end	duration		begin	end	duration
1				3			
2				4			

LOCATION

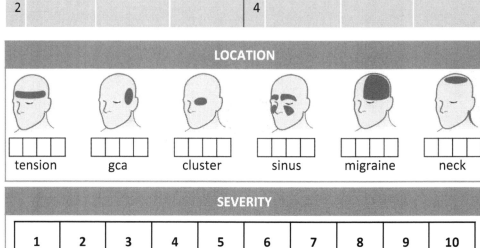

tension	gca	cluster	sinus	migraine	neck

SEVERITY

1	2	3	4	5	6	7	8	9	10

MILD   SEVERE

TRIGGERS

☐ coffee	☐ insomnia	☐ eye strain	☐ smell
☐ alcohol	☐ stress	☐ sickness	☐
☐ medication	☐ bright light	☐ travel	☐
☐ food	☐ pc/tv screen	☐ motion	☐
☐ weather	☐ reading	☐ anxiety	☐
☐ allergies	☐ noise	☐ pms	☐

RELIEF MEASURES

medication	
sleep/rest	
exercise	
Other	

DATE	

TIME

	begin	end	duration		begin	end	duration
1				3			
2				4			

LOCATION

tension	gca	cluster	sinus	migraine	neck

SEVERITY

1	2	3	4	5	6	7	8	9	10

MILD   SEVERE

TRIGGERS

☐ coffee	☐ insomnia	☐ eye strain	☐ smell
☐ alcohol	☐ stress	☐ sickness	☐
☐ medication	☐ bright light	☐ travel	☐
☐ food	☐ pc/tv screen	☐ motion	☐
☐ weather	☐ reading	☐ anxiety	☐
☐ allergies	☐ noise	☐ pms	☐

RELIEF MEASURES

medication	
sleep/rest	
exercise	
Other	

	DATE	

TIME

	begin	end	duration		begin	end	duration
1				3			
2				4			

LOCATION

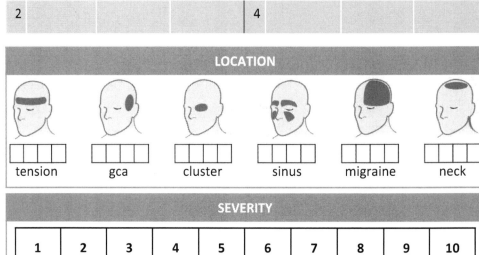

tension	gca	cluster	sinus	migraine	neck

SEVERITY

1	2	3	4	5	6	7	8	9	10

MILD   SEVERE

TRIGGERS

☐ coffee	☐ insomnia	☐ eye strain	☐ smell
☐ alcohol	☐ stress	☐ sickness	☐
☐ medication	☐ bright light	☐ travel	☐
☐ food	☐ pc/tv screen	☐ motion	☐
☐ weather	☐ reading	☐ anxiety	☐
☐ allergies	☐ noise	☐ pms	☐

RELIEF MEASURES

medication	
sleep/rest	
exercise	
Other	

DATE	

TIME

	begin	end	duration		begin	end	duration
1				3			
2				4			

LOCATION

tension	gca	cluster	sinus	migraine	neck

SEVERITY

1	2	3	4	5	6	7	8	9	10

MILD   SEVERE

TRIGGERS

☐ coffee	☐ insomnia	☐ eye strain	☐ smell
☐ alcohol	☐ stress	☐ sickness	☐
☐ medication	☐ bright light	☐ travel	☐
☐ food	☐ pc/tv screen	☐ motion	☐
☐ weather	☐ reading	☐ anxiety	☐
☐ allergies	☐ noise	☐ pms	☐

RELIEF MEASURES

medication	
sleep/rest	
exercise	
Other	

	DATE	

	begin	end	duration		begin	end	duration
1				3			
2				4			

LOCATION

tension	gca	cluster	sinus	migraine	neck

SEVERITY

1	2	3	4	5	6	7	8	9	10

MILD   SEVERE

TRIGGERS

☐ coffee	☐ insomnia	☐ eye strain	☐ smell
☐ alcohol	☐ stress	☐ sickness	☐
☐ medication	☐ bright light	☐ travel	☐
☐ food	☐ pc/tv screen	☐ motion	☐
☐ weather	☐ reading	☐ anxiety	☐
☐ allergies	☐ noise	☐ pms	☐

RELIEF MEASURES

medication	
sleep/rest	
exercise	
Other	

	DATE						

TIME

	begin	end	duration		begin	end	duration
1				3			
2				4			

LOCATION

tension	gca	cluster	sinus	migraine	neck
☐☐☐☐☐	☐☐☐☐☐	☐☐☐☐☐	☐☐☐☐☐	☐☐☐☐☐	☐☐☐☐☐

SEVERITY

1	2	3	4	5	6	7	8	9	10

MILD   SEVERE

TRIGGERS

☐ coffee	☐ insomnia	☐ eye strain	☐ smell
☐ alcohol	☐ stress	☐ sickness	☐
☐ medication	☐ bright light	☐ travel	☐
☐ food	☐ pc/tv screen	☐ motion	☐
☐ weather	☐ reading	☐ anxiety	☐
☐ allergies	☐ noise	☐ pms	☐

RELIEF MEASURES

medication	
sleep/rest	
exercise	
Other	

	DATE	

TIME

	begin	end	duration		begin	end	duration
1				3			
2				4			

LOCATION

tension	gca	cluster	sinus	migraine	neck

SEVERITY

1	2	3	4	5	6	7	8	9	10

MILD   SEVERE

TRIGGERS

- ☐ coffee
- ☐ alcohol
- ☐ medication
- ☐ food
- ☐ weather
- ☐ allergies
- ☐ insomnia
- ☐ stress
- ☐ bright light
- ☐ pc/tv screen
- ☐ reading
- ☐ noise
- ☐ eye strain
- ☐ sickness
- ☐ travel
- ☐ motion
- ☐ anxiety
- ☐ pms
- ☐ smell
- ☐
- ☐
- ☐
- ☐
- ☐

RELIEF MEASURES

medication	
sleep/rest	
exercise	
Other	

DATE	

TIME

	begin	end	duration		begin	end	duration
1				3			
2				4			

LOCATION

tension	gca	cluster	sinus	migraine	neck

SEVERITY

1	2	3	4	5	6	7	8	9	10

MILD   SEVERE

TRIGGERS

☐ coffee	☐ insomnia	☐ eye strain	☐ smell
☐ alcohol	☐ stress	☐ sickness	☐
☐ medication	☐ bright light	☐ travel	☐
☐ food	☐ pc/tv screen	☐ motion	☐
☐ weather	☐ reading	☐ anxiety	☐
☐ allergies	☐ noise	☐ pms	☐

RELIEF MEASURES

medication	
sleep/rest	
exercise	
Other	

	DATE	

TIME

	begin	end	duration		begin	end	duration
1				3			
2				4			

LOCATION

tension	gca	cluster	sinus	migraine	neck

SEVERITY

1	2	3	4	5	6	7	8	9	10

MILD　　　　　　　　　　　　　　　　　　　　　SEVERE

TRIGGERS

☐ coffee	☐ insomnia	☐ eye strain	☐ smell
☐ alcohol	☐ stress	☐ sickness	☐
☐ medication	☐ bright light	☐ travel	☐
☐ food	☐ pc/tv screen	☐ motion	☐
☐ weather	☐ reading	☐ anxiety	☐
☐ allergies	☐ noise	☐ pms	☐

RELIEF MEASURES

medication	
sleep/rest	
exercise	
Other	

DATE	

TIME

	begin	end	duration		begin	end	duration
1				3			
2				4			

LOCATION

tension	gca	cluster	sinus	migraine	neck
☐☐☐☐	☐☐☐☐	☐☐☐☐	☐☐☐☐	☐☐☐☐	☐☐☐☐

SEVERITY

1	2	3	4	5	6	7	8	9	10
MILD									SEVERE

TRIGGERS

☐ coffee	☐ insomnia	☐ eye strain	☐ smell
☐ alcohol	☐ stress	☐ sickness	☐
☐ medication	☐ bright light	☐ travel	☐
☐ food	☐ pc/tv screen	☐ motion	☐
☐ weather	☐ reading	☐ anxiety	☐
☐ allergies	☐ noise	☐ pms	☐

RELIEF MEASURES

medication	
sleep/rest	
exercise	
Other	

	DATE	

TIME

	begin	end	duration		begin	end	duration
1				3			
2				4			

LOCATION

tension	gca	cluster	sinus	migraine	neck

SEVERITY

1	2	3	4	5	6	7	8	9	10

MILD   SEVERE

TRIGGERS

☐ coffee	☐ insomnia	☐ eye strain	☐ smell
☐ alcohol	☐ stress	☐ sickness	☐
☐ medication	☐ bright light	☐ travel	☐
☐ food	☐ pc/tv screen	☐ motion	☐
☐ weather	☐ reading	☐ anxiety	☐
☐ allergies	☐ noise	☐ pms	☐

RELIEF MEASURES

medication	
sleep/rest	
exercise	
Other	

	DATE	

TIME

	begin	end	duration		begin	end	duration
1				3			
2				4			

LOCATION

tension	gca	cluster	sinus	migraine	neck

SEVERITY

1	2	3	4	5	6	7	8	9	10

MILD   SEVERE

TRIGGERS

☐ coffee	☐ insomnia	☐ eye strain	☐ smell
☐ alcohol	☐ stress	☐ sickness	☐
☐ medication	☐ bright light	☐ travel	☐
☐ food	☐ pc/tv screen	☐ motion	☐
☐ weather	☐ reading	☐ anxiety	☐
☐ allergies	☐ noise	☐ pms	☐

RELIEF MEASURES

medication	
sleep/rest	
exercise	
Other	

	DATE	

TIME

	begin	end	duration		begin	end	duration
1				3			
2				4			

LOCATION

tension	gca	cluster	sinus	migraine	neck

SEVERITY

1	2	3	4	5	6	7	8	9	10

MILD   SEVERE

TRIGGERS

☐ coffee	☐ insomnia	☐ eye strain	☐ smell
☐ alcohol	☐ stress	☐ sickness	☐
☐ medication	☐ bright light	☐ travel	☐
☐ food	☐ pc/tv screen	☐ motion	☐
☐ weather	☐ reading	☐ anxiety	☐
☐ allergies	☐ noise	☐ pms	☐

RELIEF MEASURES

medication	
sleep/rest	
exercise	
Other	

DATE	

TIME

	begin	end	duration		begin	end	duration
1				3			
2				4			

LOCATION

tension	gca	cluster	sinus	migraine	neck

SEVERITY

1	2	3	4	5	6	7	8	9	10

MILD · SEVERE

TRIGGERS

☐ coffee	☐ insomnia	☐ eye strain	☐ smell
☐ alcohol	☐ stress	☐ sickness	☐
☐ medication	☐ bright light	☐ travel	☐
☐ food	☐ pc/tv screen	☐ motion	☐
☐ weather	☐ reading	☐ anxiety	☐
☐ allergies	☐ noise	☐ pms	☐

RELIEF MEASURES

medication	
sleep/rest	
exercise	
Other	

DATE	

TIME

	begin	end	duration		begin	end	duration
1				3			
2				4			

LOCATION

tension	gca	cluster	sinus	migraine	neck

SEVERITY

1	2	3	4	5	6	7	8	9	10

MILD   SEVERE

TRIGGERS

- [ ] coffee
- [ ] alcohol
- [ ] medication
- [ ] food
- [ ] weather
- [ ] allergies
- [ ] insomnia
- [ ] stress
- [ ] bright light
- [ ] pc/tv screen
- [ ] reading
- [ ] noise
- [ ] eye strain
- [ ] sickness
- [ ] travel
- [ ] motion
- [ ] anxiety
- [ ] pms
- [ ] smell
- [ ]
- [ ]
- [ ]
- [ ]
- [ ]

RELIEF MEASURES

medication	
sleep/rest	
exercise	
Other	

DATE	

TIME

	begin	end	duration			begin	end	duration
1				|	3			
2				|	4			

LOCATION

tension	gca	cluster	sinus	migraine	neck
☐☐☐☐☐	☐☐☐☐☐	☐☐☐☐☐	☐☐☐☐☐	☐☐☐☐☐	☐☐☐☐☐

SEVERITY

1	2	3	4	5	6	7	8	9	10

MILD   SEVERE

TRIGGERS

☐ coffee	☐ insomnia	☐ eye strain	☐ smell
☐ alcohol	☐ stress	☐ sickness	☐
☐ medication	☐ bright light	☐ travel	☐
☐ food	☐ pc/tv screen	☐ motion	☐
☐ weather	☐ reading	☐ anxiety	☐
☐ allergies	☐ noise	☐ pms	☐

RELIEF MEASURES

medication	
sleep/rest	
exercise	
Other	

TIME

	begin	end	duration		begin	end	duration
1				3			
2				4			

LOCATION

tension	gca	cluster	sinus	migraine	neck

SEVERITY

1	2	3	4	5	6	7	8	9	10

MILD   SEVERE

TRIGGERS

☐ coffee	☐ insomnia	☐ eye strain	☐ smell
☐ alcohol	☐ stress	☐ sickness	☐
☐ medication	☐ bright light	☐ travel	☐
☐ food	☐ pc/tv screen	☐ motion	☐
☐ weather	☐ reading	☐ anxiety	☐
☐ allergies	☐ noise	☐ pms	☐

RELIEF MEASURES

medication	
sleep/rest	
exercise	
Other	

DATE	

TIME

	begin	end	duration		begin	end	duration
1				3			
2				4			

LOCATION

tension	gca	cluster	sinus	migraine	neck
☐☐☐☐☐	☐☐☐☐☐	☐☐☐☐☐	☐☐☐☐☐	☐☐☐☐☐	☐☐☐☐

SEVERITY

1	2	3	4	5	6	7	8	9	10

MILD   SEVERE

TRIGGERS

☐ coffee	☐ insomnia	☐ eye strain	☐ smell
☐ alcohol	☐ stress	☐ sickness	☐
☐ medication	☐ bright light	☐ travel	☐
☐ food	☐ pc/tv screen	☐ motion	☐
☐ weather	☐ reading	☐ anxiety	☐
☐ allergies	☐ noise	☐ pms	☐

RELIEF MEASURES

medication	
sleep/rest	
exercise	
Other	

TIME

	begin	end	duration		begin	end	duration
1				3			
2				4			

LOCATION

tension	gca	cluster	sinus	migraine	neck

SEVERITY

1	2	3	4	5	6	7	8	9	10

MILD   SEVERE

TRIGGERS

☐ coffee	☐ insomnia	☐ eye strain	☐ smell
☐ alcohol	☐ stress	☐ sickness	☐
☐ medication	☐ bright light	☐ travel	☐
☐ food	☐ pc/tv screen	☐ motion	☐
☐ weather	☐ reading	☐ anxiety	☐
☐ allergies	☐ noise	☐ pms	☐

RELIEF MEASURES

medication	
sleep/rest	
exercise	
Other	

		DATE				

TIME

	begin	end	duration		begin	end	duration
1				3			
2				4			

LOCATION

tension	gca	cluster	sinus	migraine	neck

SEVERITY

1	2	3	4	5	6	7	8	9	10
MILD									SEVERE

TRIGGERS

☐ coffee	☐ insomnia	☐ eye strain	☐ smell
☐ alcohol	☐ stress	☐ sickness	☐
☐ medication	☐ bright light	☐ travel	☐
☐ food	☐ pc/tv screen	☐ motion	☐
☐ weather	☐ reading	☐ anxiety	☐
☐ allergies	☐ noise	☐ pms	☐

RELIEF MEASURES

medication	
sleep/rest	
exercise	
Other	

	DATE	

TIME

	begin	end	duration		begin	end	duration
1				3			
2				4			

LOCATION

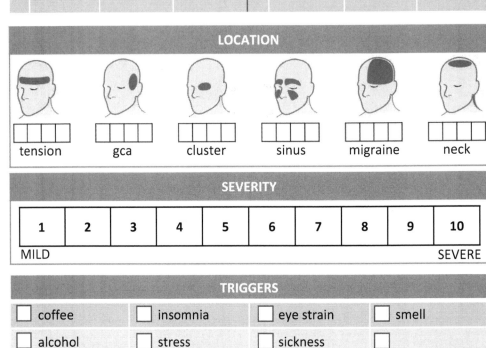

tension	gca	cluster	sinus	migraine	neck

SEVERITY

1	2	3	4	5	6	7	8	9	10

MILD   SEVERE

TRIGGERS

☐ coffee	☐ insomnia	☐ eye strain	☐ smell
☐ alcohol	☐ stress	☐ sickness	☐
☐ medication	☐ bright light	☐ travel	☐
☐ food	☐ pc/tv screen	☐ motion	☐
☐ weather	☐ reading	☐ anxiety	☐
☐ allergies	☐ noise	☐ pms	☐

RELIEF MEASURES

medication	
sleep/rest	
exercise	
Other	

DATE	

TIME

	begin	end	duration		begin	end	duration
1				3			
2				4			

LOCATION

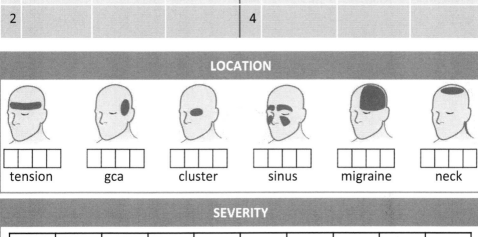

tension	gca	cluster	sinus	migraine	neck
▢▢▢▢	▢▢▢▢	▢▢▢▢	▢▢▢▢	▢▢▢▢	▢▢▢▢

SEVERITY

1	2	3	4	5	6	7	8	9	10

MILD   SEVERE

TRIGGERS

☐ coffee	☐ insomnia	☐ eye strain	☐ smell
☐ alcohol	☐ stress	☐ sickness	☐
☐ medication	☐ bright light	☐ travel	☐
☐ food	☐ pc/tv screen	☐ motion	☐
☐ weather	☐ reading	☐ anxiety	☐
☐ allergies	☐ noise	☐ pms	☐

RELIEF MEASURES

medication	
sleep/rest	
exercise	
Other	

	DATE	

TIME

	begin	end	duration		begin	end	duration
1				3			
2				4			

LOCATION

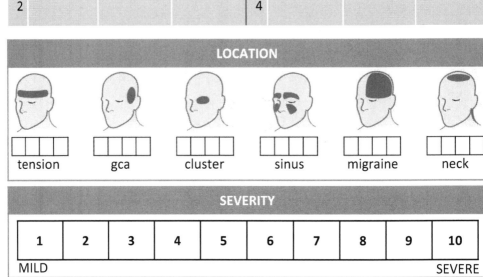

tension	gca	cluster	sinus	migraine	neck

SEVERITY

1	2	3	4	5	6	7	8	9	10

MILD   SEVERE

TRIGGERS

☐ coffee	☐ insomnia	☐ eye strain	☐ smell
☐ alcohol	☐ stress	☐ sickness	☐
☐ medication	☐ bright light	☐ travel	☐
☐ food	☐ pc/tv screen	☐ motion	☐
☐ weather	☐ reading	☐ anxiety	☐
☐ allergies	☐ noise	☐ pms	☐

RELIEF MEASURES

medication	
sleep/rest	
exercise	
Other	

	DATE	

TIME

	begin	end	duration		begin	end	duration
1				3			
2				4			

LOCATION

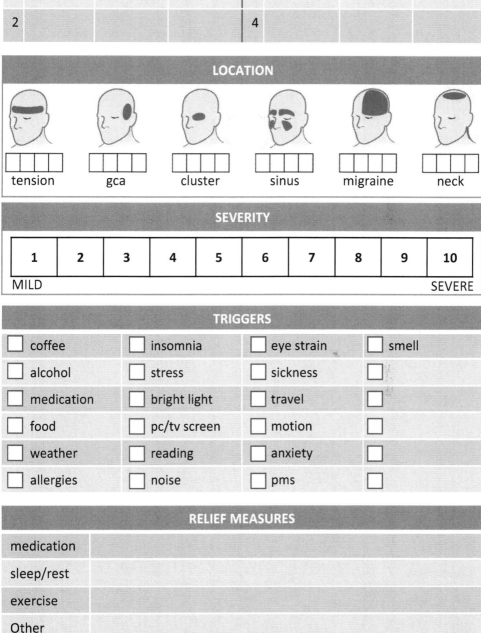

tension	gca	cluster	sinus	migraine	neck

SEVERITY

1	2	3	4	5	6	7	8	9	10

MILD   SEVERE

TRIGGERS

☐ coffee	☐ insomnia	☐ eye strain	☐ smell
☐ alcohol	☐ stress	☐ sickness	☐
☐ medication	☐ bright light	☐ travel	☐
☐ food	☐ pc/tv screen	☐ motion	☐
☐ weather	☐ reading	☐ anxiety	☐
☐ allergies	☐ noise	☐ pms	☐

RELIEF MEASURES

medication	
sleep/rest	
exercise	
Other	

		DATE				

TIME

	begin	end	duration		begin	end	duration
1				3			
2				4			

LOCATION

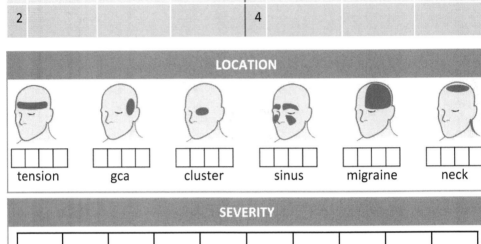

tension	gca	cluster	sinus	migraine	neck

SEVERITY

1	2	3	4	5	6	7	8	9	10

MILD SEVERE

TRIGGERS

☐ coffee	☐ insomnia	☐ eye strain	☐ smell
☐ alcohol	☐ stress	☐ sickness	☐
☐ medication	☐ bright light	☐ travel	☐
☐ food	☐ pc/tv screen	☐ motion	☐
☐ weather	☐ reading	☐ anxiety	☐
☐ allergies	☐ noise	☐ pms	☐

RELIEF MEASURES

medication	
sleep/rest	
exercise	
Other	

	DATE	

TIME

	begin	end	duration		begin	end	duration
1				3			
2				4			

LOCATION

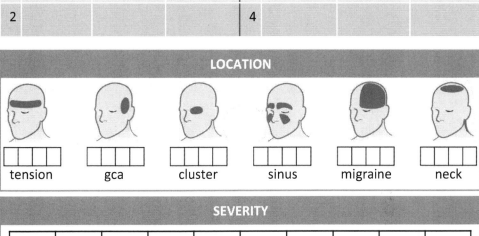

tension	gca	cluster	sinus	migraine	neck

SEVERITY

1	2	3	4	5	6	7	8	9	10

MILD | | | | | | | | | SEVERE

TRIGGERS

☐ coffee	☐ insomnia	☐ eye strain	☐ smell
☐ alcohol	☐ stress	☐ sickness	☐
☐ medication	☐ bright light	☐ travel	☐
☐ food	☐ pc/tv screen	☐ motion	☐
☐ weather	☐ reading	☐ anxiety	☐
☐ allergies	☐ noise	☐ pms	☐

RELIEF MEASURES

medication	
sleep/rest	
exercise	
Other	

	DATE	

TIME

	begin	end	duration		begin	end	duration
1				3			
2				4			

LOCATION

tension	gca	cluster	sinus	migraine	neck

SEVERITY

1	2	3	4	5	6	7	8	9	10

MILD SEVERE

TRIGGERS

☐ coffee	☐ insomnia	☐ eye strain	☐ smell
☐ alcohol	☐ stress	☐ sickness	☐
☐ medication	☐ bright light	☐ travel	☐
☐ food	☐ pc/tv screen	☐ motion	☐
☐ weather	☐ reading	☐ anxiety	☐
☐ allergies	☐ noise	☐ pms	☐

RELIEF MEASURES

medication	
sleep/rest	
exercise	
Other	

DATE	

TIME

	begin	end	duration			begin	end	duration
1				|	3			
2				|	4			

LOCATION

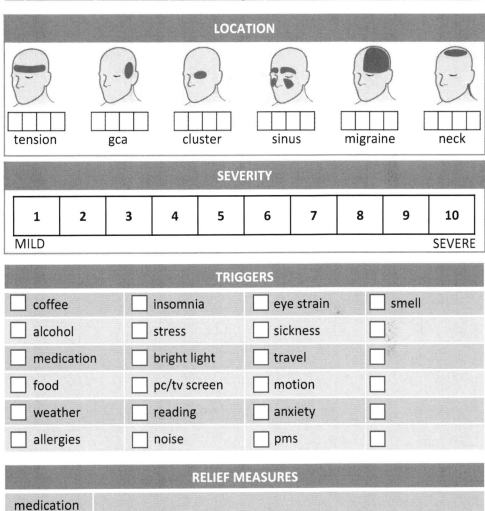

tension	gca	cluster	sinus	migraine	neck

SEVERITY

1	2	3	4	5	6	7	8	9	10

MILD   SEVERE

TRIGGERS

☐ coffee	☐ insomnia	☐ eye strain	☐ smell
☐ alcohol	☐ stress	☐ sickness	☐
☐ medication	☐ bright light	☐ travel	☐
☐ food	☐ pc/tv screen	☐ motion	☐
☐ weather	☐ reading	☐ anxiety	☐
☐ allergies	☐ noise	☐ pms	☐

RELIEF MEASURES

medication	
sleep/rest	
exercise	
Other	

			DATE		

TIME

	begin	end	duration		begin	end	duration
1				3			
2				4			

LOCATION

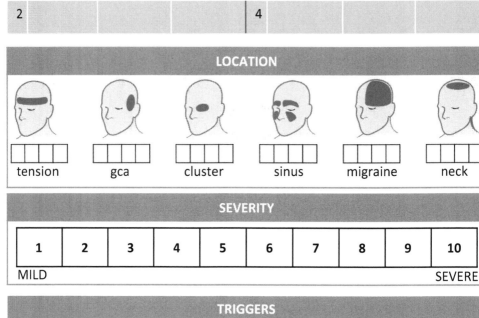

tension	gca	cluster	sinus	migraine	neck

SEVERITY

1	2	3	4	5	6	7	8	9	10

MILD   SEVERE

TRIGGERS

☐ coffee	☐ insomnia	☐ eye strain	☐ smell
☐ alcohol	☐ stress	☐ sickness	☐
☐ medication	☐ bright light	☐ travel	☐
☐ food	☐ pc/tv screen	☐ motion	☐
☐ weather	☐ reading	☐ anxiety	☐
☐ allergies	☐ noise	☐ pms	☐

RELIEF MEASURES

medication	
sleep/rest	
exercise	
Other	

DATE	

TIME

	begin	end	duration			begin	end	duration
1					3			
2					4			

LOCATION

tension	gca	cluster	sinus	migraine	neck

SEVERITY

1	2	3	4	5	6	7	8	9	10

MILD   SEVERE

TRIGGERS

☐ coffee	☐ insomnia	☐ eye strain	☐ smell
☐ alcohol	☐ stress	☐ sickness	☐
☐ medication	☐ bright light	☐ travel	☐
☐ food	☐ pc/tv screen	☐ motion	☐
☐ weather	☐ reading	☐ anxiety	☐
☐ allergies	☐ noise	☐ pms	☐

RELIEF MEASURES

medication	
sleep/rest	
exercise	
Other	

	DATE		

TIME

	begin	end	duration		begin	end	duration
1				3			
2				4			

LOCATION

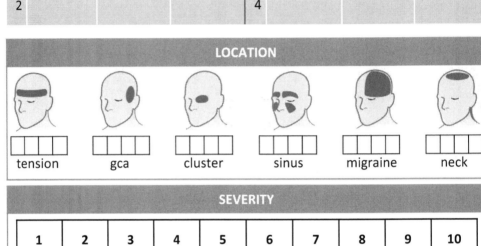

tension	gca	cluster	sinus	migraine	neck

SEVERITY

1	2	3	4	5	6	7	8	9	10

MILD　　　　　　　　　　　　　　　　　　　　　　　　　　SEVERE

TRIGGERS

☐ coffee	☐ insomnia	☐ eye strain	☐ smell
☐ alcohol	☐ stress	☐ sickness	☐
☐ medication	☐ bright light	☐ travel	☐
☐ food	☐ pc/tv screen	☐ motion	☐
☐ weather	☐ reading	☐ anxiety	☐
☐ allergies	☐ noise	☐ pms	☐

RELIEF MEASURES

medication	
sleep/rest	
exercise	
Other	

DATE	

TIME

	begin	end	duration		begin	end	duration
1				3			
2				4			

LOCATION

tension	gca	cluster	sinus	migraine	neck
☐☐☐☐	☐☐☐☐	☐☐☐☐	☐☐☐☐	☐☐☐☐	☐☐☐☐

SEVERITY

1	2	3	4	5	6	7	8	9	10

MILD   SEVERE

TRIGGERS

☐ coffee	☐ insomnia	☐ eye strain	☐ smell
☐ alcohol	☐ stress	☐ sickness	☐
☐ medication	☐ bright light	☐ travel	☐
☐ food	☐ pc/tv screen	☐ motion	☐
☐ weather	☐ reading	☐ anxiety	☐
☐ allergies	☐ noise	☐ pms	☐

RELIEF MEASURES

medication	
sleep/rest	
exercise	
Other	

	DATE		

TIME

	begin	end	duration		begin	end	duration
1				3			
2				4			

LOCATION

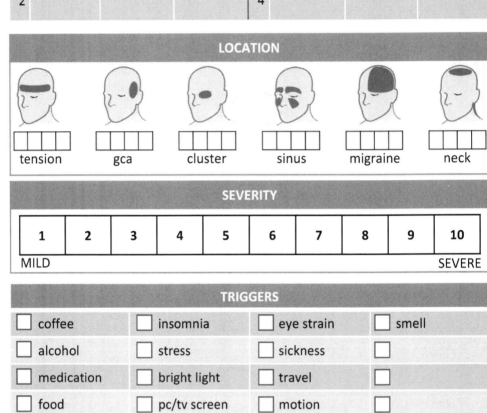

tension	gca	cluster	sinus	migraine	neck

SEVERITY

1	2	3	4	5	6	7	8	9	10

MILD   SEVERE

TRIGGERS

☐ coffee	☐ insomnia	☐ eye strain	☐ smell
☐ alcohol	☐ stress	☐ sickness	☐
☐ medication	☐ bright light	☐ travel	☐
☐ food	☐ pc/tv screen	☐ motion	☐
☐ weather	☐ reading	☐ anxiety	☐
☐ allergies	☐ noise	☐ pms	☐

RELIEF MEASURES

medication	
sleep/rest	
exercise	
Other	

DATE	

TIME

	begin	end	duration		begin	end	duration
1				3			
2				4			

LOCATION

tension	gca	cluster	sinus	migraine	neck
☐☐☐☐	☐☐☐☐	☐☐☐☐	☐☐☐☐	☐☐☐☐	☐☐☐☐

SEVERITY

1	2	3	4	5	6	7	8	9	10

MILD   SEVERE

TRIGGERS

☐ coffee	☐ insomnia	☐ eye strain	☐ smell
☐ alcohol	☐ stress	☐ sickness	☐
☐ medication	☐ bright light	☐ travel	☐
☐ food	☐ pc/tv screen	☐ motion	☐
☐ weather	☐ reading	☐ anxiety	☐
☐ allergies	☐ noise	☐ pms	☐

RELIEF MEASURES

medication	
sleep/rest	
exercise	
Other	

	DATE	

TIME

	begin	end	duration		begin	end	duration
1				3			
2				4			

LOCATION

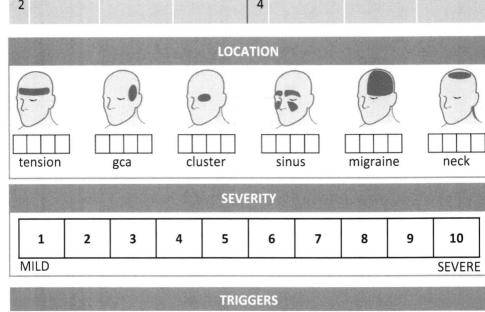

tension	gca	cluster	sinus	migraine	neck

SEVERITY

1	2	3	4	5	6	7	8	9	10

MILD   SEVERE

TRIGGERS

☐ coffee	☐ insomnia	☐ eye strain	☐ smell
☐ alcohol	☐ stress	☐ sickness	☐
☐ medication	☐ bright light	☐ travel	☐
☐ food	☐ pc/tv screen	☐ motion	☐
☐ weather	☐ reading	☐ anxiety	☐
☐ allergies	☐ noise	☐ pms	☐

RELIEF MEASURES

medication	
sleep/rest	
exercise	
Other	

	DATE		

TIME

	begin	end	duration		begin	end	duration
1				3			
2				4			

LOCATION

tension	gca	cluster	sinus	migraine	neck
☐☐☐☐☐	☐☐☐☐☐	☐☐☐☐☐	☐☐☐☐☐	☐☐☐☐☐	☐☐☐☐☐

SEVERITY

1	2	3	4	5	6	7	8	9	10

MILD   SEVERE

TRIGGERS

☐ coffee	☐ insomnia	☐ eye strain	☐ smell
☐ alcohol	☐ stress	☐ sickness	☐
☐ medication	☐ bright light	☐ travel	☐
☐ food	☐ pc/tv screen	☐ motion	☐
☐ weather	☐ reading	☐ anxiety	☐
☐ allergies	☐ noise	☐ pms	☐

RELIEF MEASURES

medication	
sleep/rest	
exercise	
Other	

		DATE		

TIME

	begin	end	duration		begin	end	duration
1				3			
2				4			

LOCATION

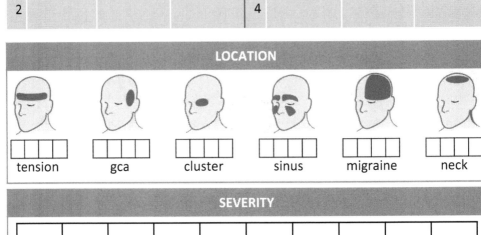

tension	gca	cluster	sinus	migraine	neck

SEVERITY

1	2	3	4	5	6	7	8	9	10

MILD   SEVERE

TRIGGERS

☐ coffee	☐ insomnia	☐ eye strain	☐ smell
☐ alcohol	☐ stress	☐ sickness	☐
☐ medication	☐ bright light	☐ travel	☐
☐ food	☐ pc/tv screen	☐ motion	☐
☐ weather	☐ reading	☐ anxiety	☐
☐ allergies	☐ noise	☐ pms	☐

RELIEF MEASURES

medication	
sleep/rest	
exercise	
Other	

DATE	

TIME

	begin	end	duration		begin	end	duration
1				3			
2				4			

LOCATION

tension	gca	cluster	sinus	migraine	neck

SEVERITY

1	2	3	4	5	6	7	8	9	10

MILD   SEVERE

TRIGGERS

☐ coffee	☐ insomnia	☐ eye strain	☐ smell
☐ alcohol	☐ stress	☐ sickness	☐
☐ medication	☐ bright light	☐ travel	☐
☐ food	☐ pc/tv screen	☐ motion	☐
☐ weather	☐ reading	☐ anxiety	☐
☐ allergies	☐ noise	☐ pms	☐

RELIEF MEASURES

medication	
sleep/rest	
exercise	
Other	

	DATE	

TIME

	begin	end	duration		begin	end	duration
1				3			
2				4			

LOCATION

tension	gca	cluster	sinus	migraine	neck
▢▢▢▢	▢▢▢▢	▢▢▢▢	▢▢▢▢	▢▢▢▢	▢▢▢▢

SEVERITY

1	2	3	4	5	6	7	8	9	10
MILD									SEVERE

TRIGGERS

☐ coffee	☐ insomnia	☐ eye strain	☐ smell
☐ alcohol	☐ stress	☐ sickness	☐
☐ medication	☐ bright light	☐ travel	☐
☐ food	☐ pc/tv screen	☐ motion	☐
☐ weather	☐ reading	☐ anxiety	☐
☐ allergies	☐ noise	☐ pms	☐

RELIEF MEASURES

medication	
sleep/rest	
exercise	
Other	

DATE	

TIME

	begin	end	duration		begin	end	duration
1				3			
2				4			

LOCATION

tension	gca	cluster	sinus	migraine	neck
☐☐☐☐	☐☐☐☐	☐☐☐☐	☐☐☐☐	☐☐☐☐	☐☐☐☐

SEVERITY

1	2	3	4	5	6	7	8	9	10

MILD   SEVERE

TRIGGERS

☐ coffee	☐ insomnia	☐ eye strain	☐ smell
☐ alcohol	☐ stress	☐ sickness	☐
☐ medication	☐ bright light	☐ travel	☐
☐ food	☐ pc/tv screen	☐ motion	☐
☐ weather	☐ reading	☐ anxiety	☐
☐ allergies	☐ noise	☐ pms	☐

RELIEF MEASURES

medication	
sleep/rest	
exercise	
Other	

	DATE	

TIME

	begin	end	duration		begin	end	duration
1				3			
2				4			

LOCATION

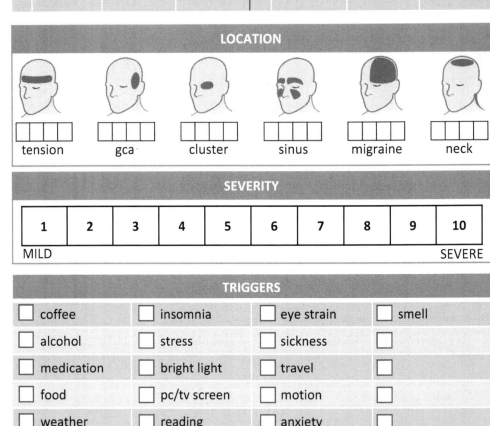

tension	gca	cluster	sinus	migraine	neck

SEVERITY

1	2	3	4	5	6	7	8	9	10

MILD   SEVERE

TRIGGERS

☐ coffee	☐ insomnia	☐ eye strain	☐ smell
☐ alcohol	☐ stress	☐ sickness	☐
☐ medication	☐ bright light	☐ travel	☐
☐ food	☐ pc/tv screen	☐ motion	☐
☐ weather	☐ reading	☐ anxiety	☐
☐ allergies	☐ noise	☐ pms	☐

RELIEF MEASURES

medication	
sleep/rest	
exercise	
Other	

DATE	

TIME

	begin	end	duration		begin	end	duration
1				3			
2				4			

LOCATION

tension	gca	cluster	sinus	migraine	neck

SEVERITY

1	2	3	4	5	6	7	8	9	10

MILD   SEVERE

TRIGGERS

☐ coffee	☐ insomnia	☐ eye strain	☐ smell
☐ alcohol	☐ stress	☐ sickness	☐
☐ medication	☐ bright light	☐ travel	☐
☐ food	☐ pc/tv screen	☐ motion	☐
☐ weather	☐ reading	☐ anxiety	☐
☐ allergies	☐ noise	☐ pms	☐

RELIEF MEASURES

medication	
sleep/rest	
exercise	
Other	

DATE	

TIME

	begin	end	duration		begin	end	duration
1				3			
2				4			

LOCATION

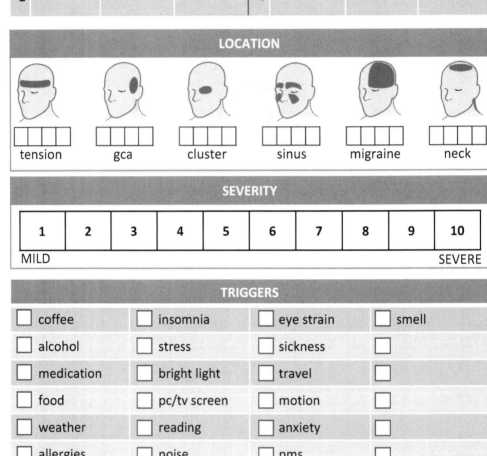

tension	gca	cluster	sinus	migraine	neck

SEVERITY

1	2	3	4	5	6	7	8	9	10

MILD   SEVERE

TRIGGERS

☐ coffee	☐ insomnia	☐ eye strain	☐ smell
☐ alcohol	☐ stress	☐ sickness	☐
☐ medication	☐ bright light	☐ travel	☐
☐ food	☐ pc/tv screen	☐ motion	☐
☐ weather	☐ reading	☐ anxiety	☐
☐ allergies	☐ noise	☐ pms	☐

RELIEF MEASURES

medication	
sleep/rest	
exercise	
Other	

DATE		

TIME

	begin	end	duration		begin	end	duration
1				3			
2				4			

LOCATION

tension	gca	cluster	sinus	migraine	neck
☐☐☐☐	☐☐☐☐	☐☐☐☐	☐☐☐☐	☐☐☐☐	☐☐☐☐

SEVERITY

1	2	3	4	5	6	7	8	9	10

MILD   SEVERE

TRIGGERS

☐ coffee	☐ insomnia	☐ eye strain	☐ smell
☐ alcohol	☐ stress	☐ sickness	☐
☐ medication	☐ bright light	☐ travel	☐
☐ food	☐ pc/tv screen	☐ motion	☐
☐ weather	☐ reading	☐ anxiety	☐
☐ allergies	☐ noise	☐ pms	☐

RELIEF MEASURES

medication	
sleep/rest	
exercise	
Other	

DATE	

TIME

	begin	end	duration		begin	end	duration
1				3			
2				4			

LOCATION

| tension | gca | cluster | sinus | migraine | neck |

SEVERITY

1	2	3	4	5	6	7	8	9	10

MILD   SEVERE

TRIGGERS

☐ coffee	☐ insomnia	☐ eye strain	☐ smell
☐ alcohol	☐ stress	☐ sickness	☐
☐ medication	☐ bright light	☐ travel	☐
☐ food	☐ pc/tv screen	☐ motion	☐
☐ weather	☐ reading	☐ anxiety	☐
☐ allergies	☐ noise	☐ pms	☐

RELIEF MEASURES

medication	
sleep/rest	
exercise	
Other	

	DATE	

TIME

	begin	end	duration		begin	end	duration
1				3			
2				4			

LOCATION

tension	gca	cluster	sinus	migraine	neck

SEVERITY

1	2	3	4	5	6	7	8	9	10

MILD · SEVERE

TRIGGERS

☐ coffee	☐ insomnia	☐ eye strain	☐ smell
☐ alcohol	☐ stress	☐ sickness	☐
☐ medication	☐ bright light	☐ travel	☐
☐ food	☐ pc/tv screen	☐ motion	☐
☐ weather	☐ reading	☐ anxiety	☐
☐ allergies	☐ noise	☐ pms	☐

RELIEF MEASURES

medication	
sleep/rest	
exercise	
Other	

	DATE	

TIME

	begin	end	duration		begin	end	duration
1				3			
2				4			

LOCATION

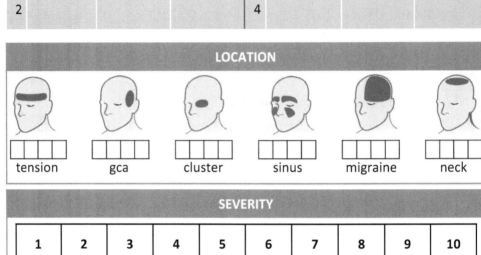

tension	gca	cluster	sinus	migraine	neck

SEVERITY

1	2	3	4	5	6	7	8	9	10

MILD   SEVERE

TRIGGERS

☐ coffee	☐ insomnia	☐ eye strain	☐ smell
☐ alcohol	☐ stress	☐ sickness	☐
☐ medication	☐ bright light	☐ travel	☐
☐ food	☐ pc/tv screen	☐ motion	☐
☐ weather	☐ reading	☐ anxiety	☐
☐ allergies	☐ noise	☐ pms	☐

RELIEF MEASURES

medication	
sleep/rest	
exercise	
Other	